Cutting Weight
101

Step-by-Step Guide to Weight Loss for Sports Performance

Carlos Y. Sumulong

Cutting Weight 101

Step-by-Step Guide to Weight Loss for Sports Performance

Publisher: CREATESPACE an Amazon Company

May 1, 2014 (Revised May, 2014)

ISBN-13: 978-0692282021 (Cutting Weight 101)

ISBN-10: 0692282025

Art direction and cover design: Kaye Denise Homecillo
Photographs copyright © 2014 by Carlos Sumulong

Manufactured in the United States of America

ISBN-10: 0692282025
ISBN-13: 978-0692282021

DEDICATION

This book is dedicated to my late mother Marilyn Sumulong with love.

I will always wake up to your beautiful music. Throughout my childhood, I watched you practice on your harp diligently, and your music remains alive to this day. You have taught me to have passion for your craft.

CONTENTS

ACKNOWLEDGEMENTS

I cannot express enough gratitude to my family for their continued support and encouragement: A special thanks to my sister Lorraine for her help and editing expertise. The completion of this project could not have been accomplished without the support of Pops, Bubs, L'Jay, and Pete. To my children Logan and Paige – thank you for allowing me time to research and write. You deserve a trip to the Harry Potter Theme Park!

I would like to recognize my first high school coach, California Wrestling Hall of Fame member Bill Gray of Oceana High School. Competing for Coach Gray for one high school season made the biggest impact in my athletic career. This is where I learned a work ethic and a never-quit attitude in the foggy hills of Pacifica, California.

My family moved to Concord, California, in my sophomore year. Although I was disappointed to move away from my friends, I soon discovered the Concord Youth Center where I was coached by Olympic and World Team Greco Roman Coaches Bill Martell and

Floyd Winters. I was exposed to high-level technique, detailed instruction and a passion for the sport. I would also like to recognize Brad Schwartz who was an inspiring coach, intense drill partner, and introduced me to the power of prayer before tournaments.

In college, National Hall of Fame member Lars Jensen coached me. Coach Jensen brought in accomplished assistant coaches, a never-ending work ethic, and tough Junior College transfers to make our room complete. He put together the toughest competition schedule against the very best Division I programs.

I would also like to acknowledge the following wrestling programs that I have been a part of. Northgate High School, Walnut Creek Wrestling Club, De LaSalle High School and the Community Youth Center (CYC).

Finally, I would like to thank my loving wife, Heather. Your encouragements when the times got rough are much appreciated. It was a great have your knowledge base and assistance in developing the cutting weight 101 method, meal plans, and structure of the book.

INTRODUCTION

Let me start off by introducing myself. My name is Carlos Sumulong. I am the co-owner of VQ Fit Pros (Strength & Conditioning Company), a Certified Strength Conditioning Specialist with the National Strength Conditioning Association(CSCS/NSCA), and a passionate wrestling coach. Above all else, I am a husband, a father, and brother.

I have been a wrestler since I stepped inside the Oceana High School wrestling room at the age of ten. I started off with minimal success in middle school and played a lot of recreation sports, such as football and basketball. During middle school I developed a strong desire for the challenging sport of wrestling. In my sophomore year in high school, I decided to specialize in wrestling and take my sport to another level. I loved the discipline and courage components of an individual sport. There is a strong brotherhood in the wrestling community because of the relationships formed from the grueling practices, road trips, and the work ethic necessary for success. I find it remarkable how participating in one of the oldest sports known to mankind makes such a huge mark on your soul.

I was fortunate enough to grow up with great coaches as mentors. Many of them happened to be Olympic and World Team coaches who have been inducted into the National Wrestling Hall of Fame. My wrestling coaches have helped shaped me into the man I am today. These coaches contributed selflessly toward my development as an athlete and made the sport fun!

Working with passionate coaches helped me achieve a rewarding and successful career in high school. After being recruited by many colleges, I decided to wrestle for San Francisco State University. I finished my career as NCAA DII All American, team captain for the 1997 NCAA DII National Champion Team, and won the Arete Award for excellence in academics and athletics. In 2009 I was honored to be inducted to the SFSU NCAA

Athletic Hall Of Fame and I am forever grateful to the selection committee and Coach Lars Jensen.

Following a rewarding college athletic career I decided to work for myself and start a strength conditioning consulting company with my wife Heather. We founded VQ Fit Pros in 1998. Being self-employed immediately out of college was very challenging. I was very fortunate to meet incredible clients early on who became my business mentors. We won Diablo Magazine's Best Personal Trainer of the East Bay for two consecutive years.

Alongside my personal training career, I began coaching wrestling at the high school level. Many of my athletes went on to become successful college wrestlers, MMA athletes, and successful businessmen. After my son showed an interest in the sport, I decided to start a youth club team. When competing at state and national level tournaments, there are always a handful of wrestlers who want to cut weight and get the edge.

Cutting Weight. There! I said it. That big dark cloud that makes so many people cringe. Making weight and cutting weight are words that bring up negative images of high school wrestlers running around their school in garbage bags, spitting in cups, and missing several meals during the week. I have seen several good athletes quit the sport of wrestling because they did not like cutting weight.

I have been coaching wrestling since 1997 and have seen several wrestling diets. Most of the literature passed out to young wrestlers will have a long list of healthy food for wrestlers to eat. The problem is that they lack a true plan of action for a healthy weight loss during the week going into a weigh-in. When I cut weight as a high school and college athlete, I had no idea what I was doing. I sampled several quick fix diets and tried to implement them, but I would still resort to unhealthy weight cuts. If you named all of the unhealthy weight loss methods, I probably did most of them.

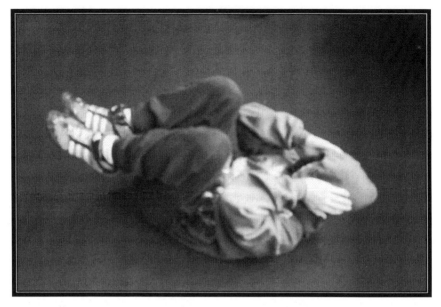

My college roommates would often find me cutting weight in this position.

My personal record in college was a water weight loss of 15 pounds in one day for a dual meet against UC Davis. This was a common practice for college wrestlers before weight management programs were implemented. The hydration testing methods that are now required in high school and college wrestling are designed to prevent big weight cuts.

Let me clarify that this was mostly water weight loss. Being an exercise science major, I volunteered to do the hydrostatic body fat test and Bod Pod (Body Composition Measurement) in our college exercise physiology lab. Results showed that I only had four percent body fat. Essential body fat is three percent.

This was extremely unhealthy because there was no body fat left to lose and I would just waste away essential lean body mass. I had very little body fat and made the extreme sacrifice to make a lower weight class, so I could make the starting line up. I made weight the night before and competed the next day twenty pounds heavier and won a Conference Championship. These were the extreme weight cuts that happened during my college days. I'm happy to say that things are much different today, due to the changes in weigh ins and hydration testing. I do not recommend the extreme methods that I practiced during my career.

I would repeat this unhealthy routine every week throughout my college-wrestling career. Cutting a lot of weight as a wrestler was sometimes like wearing a badge of honor similar to getting cauliflower ear from spending hours on the mat. As a college student, I would eat the disgusting dorm food and then work out like a madman after practice to get my weight down.

Fifteen years after my last college match, my career is still involved with a different type of weight loss. I deal with the daily weight loss goals and health concerns of my clients. I have seen every diet, calorie counter and diet pill. I have worked with many Registered Dieticians and helped implement solid nutrition plans for my clients. However, even with sound nutrition plans many of my clients still want to try the quick-fix fad diets designed to reach short-term weight loss goals. I monitor their body fat, food journals, and check their weight before every session. As a health professional I have discovered that many wrestlers, coaches, and parents lack a true plan for a healthy weight loss.

I have helped numerous wrestlers cut weight in a healthy way. It has been my dream to write a book about my experiences with cutting weight as an athlete and a coach. My mission is to give everyone the necessary tools to reach their weight loss goals in a safe and efficient way.

Cutting Weight 101 is a book that maps out an effective weight loss plan for athletes in every age group. My plan is specifically directed toward athletes in the 9-24%

body fat category. If you are 7-8% body fat or lower, you can focus on eating more nutrient dense calories and putting on more lean muscle mass for your weight class. There is a method to cutting weight. You can make weight and still feel strong going into a tournament. Anyone can follow this plan and apply it toward their weight loss goals. This book will help wrestlers make weight properly. It will also help anyone else that wants a jump-start to his or her weight loss goals. Just remember that wrestlers work out between 10-14 hours a week, which is why they lose body fat and water weight so quickly. I hope you pick up some great tips from this book, avoid unhealthy methods, and embrace the daily process for reaching your goal!

CHAPTER 1

WHY SHOULD I CUT?

The American sports society is a culture addicted to winning, dominating, and measuring self-worth on win-loss records. It is a culture that will always come up with creative avenues to get a competitive advantage. "Cutting weight," a term associated with weight loss in combat sports that require weight divisions in order to compete, is one such avenue.

Every season ultra-competitive coaches ask wrestlers to drop to a lower weight class for their team. It happens in youth football as well. Players are often asked to drop weight to compete in the older lighter division. These ultra competitive coaches always want the best athletes in their line-up. They are looking for their strongest team possible. They are looking to increase their team's chances and walk out victorious after the game. It's all about repetitions, playing time, and getting the edge on the competition.

The cutting weight mindset encourages the athlete to go down to a lower weight class and have an opportunity to be stronger and a little bit bigger than his or her opponent. Being bigger, faster, and stronger than your opponent can sometimes give you the advantage you need to secure victory.

It is worth noting that the governing athletic associations such as the National Federation of State High School Associations (NFHS) and the NCAA want skill and technique, not rapid weight cutting, to determine the wrestler's tool for success.

Over the last several years, the NFHS Wrestling Rules Committee has adopted rules that attempt to discourage wrestlers from losing extreme amounts of weight. The most significant rules include:

- Requiring each wrestler to establish a certified minimum weight before January 15.
- Prohibiting a wrestler from wrestling more than one weight class above the certified weight without recertifying at a higher weight.
- Recommending body fat measurements and hydration levels in establishing a minimum certified weight.
- Prohibiting the use of sweatboxes, vinyl suits, diuretics or other artificial means of quick weight reduction.
- Permitting wrestlers to have a two-pound growth allowance.
- Requiring shoulder-to-shoulder weigh-ins one hour before the start of a dual meet and two hours before tournaments.

The Rules Committee made a strong statement in revising the weigh-in procedure and emphasized the importance of safety in urging wrestlers to wrestle as close to their natural weight as possible.

The NCAA weight management program states that a sensible alternative to dehydration weight loss is outlined in the original established principles of the NCAA weight management program:

- Enhance safety and competitive equity.
- Minimize incentives for rapid weight loss.
- Emphasize competition, not weight control; and
- Implement practical, effective and enforceable guidelines.

The goals of the NCAA weight management program remain the same as when it was originally established in 1998:

- Establish weight classes that better reflect the collegiate wrestling population.
- Establish a permanent healthy weight class early in the season with time to achieve it safely.
- Establish weigh-ins as close to the match as possible and a random draw for weight class order.
- Eliminate the tools used to accomplish rapid dehydration.

Even though the wrestling culture is slowly changing, weight cutting is still very much alive. My goal in this book is to help athletes lose a few pounds the right way. If you are a smaller athlete and your opponent of equal or greater ability dropped four pounds to make weight, you might find yourself in a slight strength disadvantage. I have experienced both ends of the spectrum from being the smaller guy and losing to a bigger opponent and being the bigger guy who dropped a few extra pounds to get the win. This competitive scenario will always breed a need to "lose a few pounds" and look for small advantages over opponents.

The power of the human will to compete and the drive to excel beyond the body's normal capabilities is most beautifully demonstrated in the arena of sport.
-Aimee Mullins

Dedicated athletes have a burning desire to do the extra workouts to outwork the competition. There is no better feeling than getting your arm raised after a wrestling match or helping your team win with a game winning play.

Sports also teach young athletes how to deal with adversity. Wrestlers learn how to deal with extreme adversity from pre-competition jitters, stepping on the big stage with a large audience, and going against an intimidating opponent by yourself.

Participating in sports not only develops your character, it reveals it. How do you deal with a loss? Can you lose with dignity, or do you play the blame game with coaches or teammates? I struggle sometimes with this question, but looking at the big picture, my job as a coach is to develop strong, hardworking, and dependable individuals.

Coaches can learn a lot from looking at the grand scheme of their program and not be short sided and focus so much on just the winning results. It is the short-sided mentality of a few coaches that encourages cheating, the quick fix short cut, and unhealthy methods in making weight.

Sports teach all participants that there are no short cuts. Hard work is the prerequisite and building block to success on the field. As a coach I've seen many athletes go through several years of losing before they taste a winning season. This type of athlete is comfortable with adversity and is a mentally tough individual. These athletes have adapted to the grueling process of daily training, dealing with losing, and will carry the work ethic they developed from their sport for the rest of their life. It is very satisfying to coach young athletes who are coachable, have clear goals, consistent motivation, and then to see them ultimately accomplish their big dream goals.

> *Goals are dreams with deadlines.*
> *-Diana Scharf*

"Why should I cut?" Wrestlers cut weight because they want the advantage of being the stronger athlete over their opponent or to earn a spot on the starting line-up. Many nutritionists and physicians are completely against quick weight loss for any sport. However many athletes are still looking to get an advantage over their opponents.

Today's young athletes have a difficult time distinguishing the difference between sound nutrition principles and dated methods of quick water weight loss. Many young wrestlers will do a starvation diet a five days before weigh-ins and sweat out the last two to three pounds an hour before weigh-ins. I remember seeing a young athlete try laxatives and running in garbage bags in order to make weight for his football game.

I do not recommend cutting weight for wrestling at the elementary school age. Until the athlete has had a few years of competition and embraces the challenging demands for the sport, most young athletes are not mentally mature enough for the discipline required in following a diet for weight loss. I've seen many young wrestlers burn out before high school because they cut a lot of weight every month from 3rd grade to 8th grade. There are a lot of individuals that are not on their high school team right now that have won multiple youth state and national medals. Avoid cutting weight at a young age.

For a large number of overweight teenage participants, losing weight is highly recommended because many are showing up with high body fat test, scoring between 16-

30%. The obese athletes have several health risks associated with their current diet and end up having the true success stories in the wrestling season. They have real world results in weight loss because of their discipline, dedication, and life changing mentality to transform their body by grinding it out in one of the toughest sports to participate in.

The Cutting Weight 101 method is designed for high school age athletes or adults who need to make weight at a lower weight class. An example would be a 18 year-old wrestler who walks around at 157 and wants to compete at 152 pounds. He is in the middle of the 160-pound and 152-pound weight class. If he competes at 160 pounds, there is a good chance that he may compete against someone who dropped from 163 pounds. A strong 163 pounder versus a 157 pounder can be a tough match for the smaller athlete. The five-pound difference is significant when it comes to strength, speed, and explosiveness.

By joining wrestling, martial arts, or any other contact sport, the foundation of discipline and hard work in training puts an athlete in the best shape of his life because these sports are so physically and mentally challenging. These athletes easily burn over 500-1000 calories each practice. Combat sports and mixed martial art workouts offer a high metabolic demand on the body. By midseason most wrestlers have burned off significant body fat. They have also certified their lowest weight class for the season and are following NHSCA weight loss guidelines.

If a wrestler wants to lose 4-6 pounds for the league finals, then this is the book that will map out an easy, healthy, smart system to get down to the athlete's optimum weight class. Cutting weight for sport is a personal choice and should be an open discussion between the coach, parents, and athlete. Once the athlete, parents, and coach decide to go down to a lower weight class, they should map out the plan of action to reach the lower weight class.

It is also important to get a good estimate on your real weight. "Morning Weigh-in" is a great way to estimate your real weight. Check your weight after you go to the bathroom and track your data in your journal. After a week of journaling, you will see get a good idea of your

CHAPTER 2

OLD SCHOOL METHODS

When I first started wrestling in high school as a freshman, I showed a lot of promise by beating out a senior to get the starting varsity spot. Immediately after winning the challenge match on Thursday, I stepped on the scale and saw that I was 8 pounds over for the weekend tournament. I was expected to lose 8 pounds in order to make weight for the upcoming varsity tournament on Saturday. I did not question it. I felt obligated to my coach, and to be honest, he scared the living daylights out of me. This was the first time I had to cut weight in my wrestling career. I did not have a plan on how I was going to lose the weight. I just knew that I had to run a lot and sweat a ton.

Thus began the painful process of making the cut from 123 to 114 pounds. I was already at a low body fat and had to find a way to lose eight pounds of water weight before Saturday's weigh-in. My older brother was also a wrestler, so he helped me with my first cut. I ran for two and a half hours Friday night. It was sixty degrees, windy and foggy. This is typical weather in the coastal community of Pacifica, California. I had to put on three layers of sweatshirts, sweat pants, and I put on a sauna suit underneath the layers before my long weight cut run. Running long and not eating or drinking the night before weigh-ins was very painful and taxing on my body. After hours of running in layers, I felt weak, dehydrated, and really wanted to grab a drink from the refrigerator.

Saturday morning came. Since we did not have a home scale, and I just stepped on the school scale that morning hoping I would make weight. There I was standing on the scale, a sucked up fourteen-year-old kid, every abdominal muscle visible, pronounced cheekbones, and not an ounce of energy left in my body. I stepped on the scale and heard a small clink sound indicating that I made weight. I did it! My first weight cut! Hours of running, sacrifice, and having the discipline to stay away from food and water until I made weight!

Despite all that hard work, I did not win a match in my first varsity tournament and lost to older and more experienced opponents. Little did I know that these old school methods were unhealthy and would leave me feeling tired during tournaments and dual meets.

In my sophomore year in high school, I experimented cutting weight with saunas and steam rooms inside local gyms and fitness centers. Each session would consist of several 10 minute sessions inside the sauna, getting a good sweat, and hopefully losing those last two painful pounds. After each sauna session, I would make weight and rehydrate immediately. This is a short cut method to cutting weight.

There was a big problem with this method of cutting weight. I had no energy on the mat. I always felt drained during my matches because the sauna sucked out valuable electrolytes that my body needed in order to perform at a high level. Your body is meant to operate at 98.7F. A core temperature reaching up to 105F can constitute medical help. Heat stroke can develop when the body is unable to get rid of the excess heat being produced. I experienced nausea, dizziness, and hyperventilation from my sauna use. Dehydration and salt depletion from the sauna can cause tiredness, cramping, and loss of performance.

Starvation diets and cutting out water a day before weigh-ins was another popular method that I practiced weekly in my high school career. Every Monday, I would starve myself and not eat lunch or dinner four days prior to my weigh-in. This starvation diet also had me feeling tired and drained the entire week. I practiced at half strength, performed at a low level, and was putting my body through hell. I didn't know any other way so I continued to torture myself with these "old school" methods of weight loss.

As I moved into college, I quickly found out I was entering a whole new level of weight cutting. The cutting weight culture for college wrestling during my time was absolutely nuts! I competed in the early 90's, before hydration testing, body fat testing, and NWCA weight certification. I have a small frame and competed in the lightest weight class in college. I started the preseason at 158 and got down to 142 pounds with 4% body fat.

The hardest weight cut that my body had to endure in my entire wrestling career was for the Conference Championships and the NCAA Western Regionals. I started the week at 142 pounds and made weight at the 118 pound division. There were countless hours of running and starving all week. The last day was pure torture where I was riding a bike in the steam room with layers on. It felt like I spent half the day on the bike. This routine was common among most college wrestlers at that time. I was so dehydrated that it took me half a day to lose three tenths of a pound. I was stuck at 118.3 all day, and then I finally squeezed the water out of my body by doing jumping jacks in the sauna. I did the impossible and made weight at 118.0 pounds. I rehydrated and carb loaded that night.

When I competed at the Championships the following day, I felt drained in the semi-finals, and had an unremarkable tournament performance taking 3rd place. I missed qualifying for the National tournament and was absolutely devastated. Unfortunately, this was my weight loss routine throughout my entire college career. I bumped up a weight class and competed in the 126 pound division for the next three years, but I was still cutting from 144-146 pounds at 4% body fat.

I wish I knew then what I know now about nutrition, dehydration and weight loss. The American College of Sports Medicine uses the following standards for body fat. Essential body fat for men is 2-5%, athletes 6-13%, fitness 14-17%, and 18-24% average range. Essential body fat for women is 10-13%, athletes 14-20%, fitness 21-24% fitness, and 25-31% average range.

I was burning lean body mass at 4% body fat, overtraining, and feeling mentally fatigued from the daily abuse of cutting weight improperly. My body was starting to break down in the middle of the season. This severe weight cutting routine led to several injuries during the season. My power output was affected, and my injuries forced me to miss valuable competition time. I was missing the key component of good nutrition. I trained hard, was mentally and physically tough, but the body needs to have healthy cells in order to thrive in a brutal combat sport.

My story of cutting weight is a perfect example of how not to cut weight to reach a lower weight class. This is the old school way of cutting weight before the new rules and guidelines were set forth by the NHSCA. Unfortunately, to this day many misinformed coaches and parents are still practicing many of the old school methods. People don't know any better. I see it all the time. Kids are still doing starvation diets, not hydrating properly, and wearing garbage bags or sauna suits in a hot wrestling room to cut their water weight.

The NCAA now has the following guidelines of improper weight loss for participating wrestlers.

PROHIBITED PRACTICES

The use of the following practices is prohibited for any purpose:

1. Vapor impermeable suits (e.g., rubber suits or rubberized nylon);
2. Similar devices used for dehydration;
3. Saunas (even off campus);

4. Steam rooms (even off campus);

5. Wrestling room over 75 degrees at start of practice;

6. Hot boxes;

7. Laxatives (non-prescribed); Diuretics

8. Emetics;

9. Excessive food and fluid restriction;

10. Self-induced vomiting;

11. Artificial means of re-hydration (i.e., intravenous hydration).

Violators of these rules will be suspended for the competition(s) for which the weigh-in is intended. A second violation would result in suspension for the remainder of the season. Coaches aware of these violations are also held to these same penalties.

The old school methods listed above are clearly practices that should be avoided by all athletes. From personal experience, the daily grind of cutting over ten pounds a week before every tournament negatively affected my sports performance. The starvation diet robbed my body of essential nutrients. I over-trained my body with minimal fuel, which led to an increase of injuries.

I hope athletes can learn from my mistakes and avoid the old school methods of starvation diets, saunas, fluid restriction, and the use of diuretics. I wrote this book to help athletes compete at their optimal weight class with healthy nutrition. It is really a very simple formula. Follow this plan, watch the weight drop off, stay hydrated and nourished, and perform at your highest level!

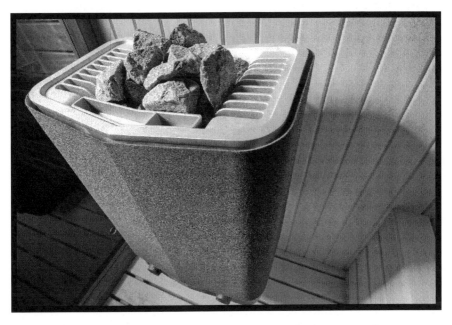

Sauna use while dehydrated is dangerous and can affect sports performance.

CHAPTER 3

COMMON MISTAKES

I have seen and adopted many unhealthy habits related to weight cutting in my thirty years as an athlete and coach. Many of these habits are created in part by a misinformed group of coaches, athletes and parents who endorse old school methods of weight cutting to young athletes. For years the culture of wrestling accepted extreme measures of water weight loss and starvation diets.

Starting a weight cut without a safe and healthy system usually involves a lot of guesswork that can leave the athlete drained, frustrated, and confused. Below is a list of common mistakes people make during their weight cut process:

1. **Wearing heavy layers during practice early in the week to lose water weight.** Losing water weight early in the week leads to early dehydration and poor practices leading up to your competition. This is a common scene in many wrestling rooms. I've seen many wrestlers wear several long sleeved layers, sweat pants, and a beanie while they drill and wrestle live in a hot wrestling room. Many of them think that this is an effective method to getting their weight down. Wearing several layers early in your training cycle will definitely lead to water weight loss, but doing this early in the week leads to water retention. This makes the last day of weight cutting difficult because there is nothing left to sweat out. You want to be fully hydrated going into to your last practice before weigh-ins. By doing this, you can drop an easy 1-2 pounds at the practice the night before you need to weigh in.

The following page displays a picture of the traditional wrestler weight cut outfit. Layers of shirts under a sweatshirt, tucked into sweat pants, socks over sweat pants, and a hood covering their head in order to keep the sweat going. Some wrestlers believe they will get a jump-start in their weight loss for the week. Stop torturing yourself early in the week and focus on having a great practices. Practice and drill in a t-shirt and compression shorts early in the week.

Heavy layered cardio and wearing long sleeve t-shirts during practice is a common practice with wrestlers and mixed martial art athletes. Save the layers until your last workout before weigh-ins. If weigh-ins are Saturday morning, you can put on a sweat shirt and sweat pants on your two mile run Friday night. After your run, practice in a t-shirt and shorts. If you find the need to put extra layers on early in the week, then you probably picked a weight class that is too low for you.

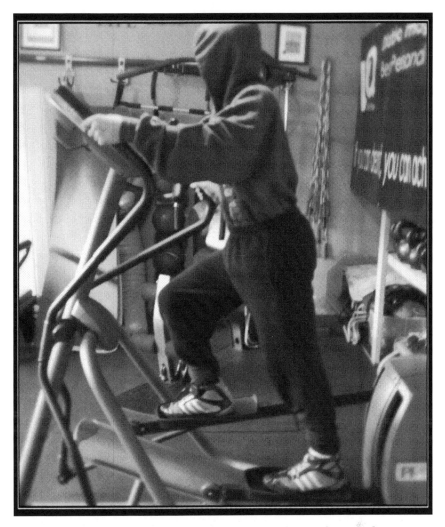

Avoid heavy layered cardio early in the week.

2. **Starvation Diet.** Skipping meals during the week means running low on energy during school, practice, and compromised power output during competition. When you are in starvation mode, your body uses stored glucose and fat, eventually

leading the body to metabolize muscle, tissues and organs in an attempt to get nutrients. Nutrient deficiencies can lead to dizziness, fatigue, and inefficient immune system. These symptoms can make workouts difficult, affect motivation, and break down important lean muscle mass. I can remember starving myself to make weight. It was difficult to focus in school. I lost significant lean body mass and felt like I was running on empty during the crucial third round in matches.

3. **Cutting out water early in the week.** This leads to lethargy, and dehydration. The outcome of this is low energy during school, practice, and compromised power output during competition. You need to stay hydrated during your training cycle.

4. **Use of caffeine pills, high-energy drinks, and pre-workout supplements.** These quick energy stimulants can cause a quick rise in blood pressure, energy crashes, cause difficulty sleeping,

and digestive problems. Please do not put this type of stress on your body.

5. **Use of saunas, steam rooms, and hot tubs for quick water weight loss.** The human body responds to heat by expanding the blood vessels, which can then deliver more blood to the skin, where extra heat escapes. Cooling comes from the evaporation of sweat, which begins when the core blood temperature rises by a degree. As your core temperature rises, blood pressure drops, heart rate goes up and the heart will pump as much as three times more blood. When you spend over 15-20 minutes in a hot sauna, the body will lose fluids and hinder the skin's ability to sweat and the heart's ability to keep up with demand. As the air in the sauna grows more humid, your sweat will stop evaporating, eliminating its ability to cool. Combined with the drop in blood pressure, dehydration and severe heat exhaustion, this can lead to fainting. Heart attacks can also ensue. Proteins can become denatured, causing a complete shutdown of the kidneys or other organ systems.

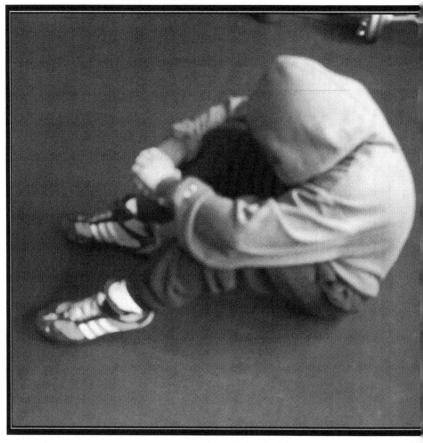

Exercising while dehydrated can lead to poor practices.

6. **Cutting out carbohydrates early in the week.** This can leave the athlete feeling fatigued, light headed, and sluggish during school and practice. This method early in the week will play havoc on blood sugar levels, causing many athletes to hit the wall. Carbohydrate is your energy source. Just make sure to stay away from

processed carbohydrates like cookies, crackers and granola bars. You want to get most of your carbs from fruit, vegetables, nuts and beans.

7. **Eating junk food.** The high fat, sodium, and sugar in junk food makes for a difficult weight cut. Trying to burn off a cheese pizza and soda from the cafeteria can take a long time to burn off. Many teenagers eat 50% of their weekly calories from fast food and high sugar drinks. The consumption of these foods will do little for your energy. This diet prevents athletes from attaining peak energy levels.

8. **Not eating enough high fiber foods.** Fiber has several health benefits and also makes fat less likely to be absorbed in your body. High fiber diets promote satiety (fullness), which is a great asset to a weight loss program. You want to feel full and enjoy the benefits of a nutrient dense diet.

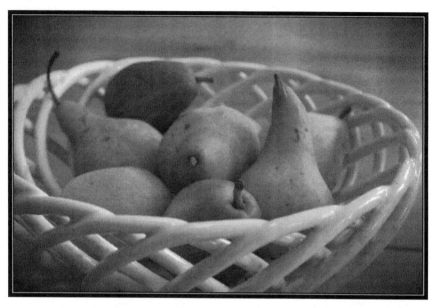

You can get up to three grams of fiber for a piece of fruit.

9. **Use of laxatives**. Many wrestlers use laxatives as a quick solution to weight loss. Frequent bowel movements caused by laxatives give people a false sense of weight loss from water. This can be unhealthy for your body and can create many unpleasant side effects. Common side effects include stomach cramping, nausea, vomiting, and diarrhea. Laxatives can cause a loss of important electrolytes to the body. Electrolyte imbalance can lead to muscle fatigue, dehydration, dizziness, and fainting. I was coaching peewee football practice a few years ago and noticed one my

players running to bathroom every five minutes. He spent half of the practice in the bathroom and was barely on the field. When I asked him about his frequent bathroom trips, he mentioned that his dad gave him laxatives so he can lose weight for the upcoming game. He was over by seven pounds and had to make the weight to be eligible to play. I then took him under my wing and taught him how to cut weight properly. I gave his dad a simple meal plan to follow and made sure they eliminated their drive thru habits. He was able to make weight and had a great year of youth football.

CHAPTER 4

NEW MINDSET

When it comes to losing weight for sports, Cutting Weight 101 offers a new mindset that can actually help improve sports performance. Every season new wrestlers sign up for their high school team, learn the challenges of the sport, quit and never return because of old school methods of cutting weight. They quit because they don't like having to watch their diet and hydration. It's already difficult to keep kids on the team because wrestling is one of the toughest combat sports to learn.

Discipline is a prerequisite for weight loss - discipline in your physical conditioning and more importantly discipline in your diet. The Cutting Weight 101 mindset involves doing the opposite of the old school methods.

The new mindset will require a healthy lifestyle of eating clean and green, keeping hydrated, and proper nutrient timing after tough workouts. This lifestyle involves bringing home nutrient dense food from the grocery. Do your grocery run at the beginning of the week so you set yourself up for success. Get the junk food out of your house to eliminate any temptations. You can use the super foods list provided in this book to give you the proper antioxidant boost for sports performance.

The mindset also involves re-training the coaching staff, student athletes, and parents. The entire team should be informed about the disadvantages of the old school methods of cutting weight through starvation diets and rapid water weight reduction practices. You can eat healthy and drink all week and still make weight for your upcoming match! It is very important that you are all on the same page.

Don't expect a magic pill or quick shortcuts. Making weight in a safe way will still require discipline, dedication, and accountability. Grueling practices will provide a high metabolic demand on the system, enhancing accelerated body fat reduction. Staying disciplined in your diet and doing extra cardio workouts to get your weight down will test the wrestler's will power. Will you stick to the healthy eating plan or give in to the high sodium high sugar meals that surround you?

There are a lot of wrestlers who have great workouts every day, but go home to a house full of junk food, frozen dinners and high sugar drinks. The goal for the season is to eat clean 75% of the time, make the right choices when you shop for groceries, and fill your kitchen with lots of healthy snacks, fruits, and vegetables. Slowly eliminate the frozen food, ice cream, and frozen pizza from your refrigerator. Clean out your pantry and throw out the crackers, cookies, and chips. It is easier to follow this method if the entire family is compliant and on board with the weight loss goal.

Here is a sample list of smart choices when going grocery shopping.

Easy Grocery Shopping Tips

1. Plan ahead. It will take a few minutes to make a list of healthy meals for the week.

2. When making your list for the week, use the super foods list in this chapter. This list contains food with a high ORAC value (unit of measurement for antioxidants).

3. Eat before going to the store. Don't grocery shop when you are hungry. You are more likely to buy high sugar and fatty foods on an empty stomach.

4. Shop the perimeter of the store, looking through fruits, vegetables, lean meat, fish, and poultry. The center aisles are filled with processed junk food items.

5. Shop for color. Avoid buying white - sugar, dairy, and processed food.

6. Shop organic, but don't replace eating organic food over eating produce.

7. Read labels and avoid processed foods that contain hydrogenated fats and oils. You should avoid crackers, cookies, chips, etc.

8. Look for low fat protein: Chicken, turkey, pork, fish, and tofu. Organic is best.

9. Look for complex carbohydrates that stimulate the least amount of insulin - barley, oatmeal, apples, pears, grapefruit, grapes, peaches, and whole wheat - so you can avoid a blood sugar crash that happens after a high sugar meal.

ORAC Value

An ORAC (Oxygen Radical Absorbance Capacity) unit is a unit of measurement for antioxidants developed by the National Institute on Aging in the National Institutes of Health (NIH). It is believed that foods higher on the ORAC scale will more effectively neutralize free radicals. Free radicals are produced during exercise.

Whether elite athletes or recreational exercisers should take antioxidant supplements remains controversial. However, it is important that those who exercise regularly ingest foods rich in antioxidants. Free radical damage during exercise induces fatigue, reduces muscle power and prolongs muscle recovery. Therefore, it has been theorized by sports nutrition researchers that increasing antioxidant consumption prior to exercise sessions might help reduce free radical damage and the associated fatigue/performance/recovery effects. A number of the antioxidants tested by researchers have shown promising results toward exercise recovery and reduced muscle fatigue scores. Here is our super foods list and their ORAC value.

Super Foods List

(ORAC Value Score=Antioxidant Capacity)

Fruits antioxidant values

1. Prunes 5770
2. Acai Berry 3800
3. Raisins 2830
4. Blue Berries 2400
5. Black Berries 2036
6. Cranberries 1750
7. Strawberries 1540
8. Pomegranates 1245
9. Raspberries 1220
10. Plums 940
11. Oranges 750
12. Red Grapes 739
13. Cherries 670
14. Cantaloupe 252
15. Banana 221

16. Apple 218

17. Apricots 164

18. Pear 134

Vegetables antioxidant value

1. Kale 1770

2. Spinach/raw 1260

3. Brussels Sprouts 980

4. Alfalfa Sprouts 930

5. Spinach/Steamed 909

6. Broccoli Florets 890

7. Beets 841

8. Red Bell Pepper 713

9. Onion 450

10. Corn 400

11. Eggplant 390

12. Cauliflower 377

13. Sweet Potato 301

14. Carrots 207

15. String Beans 201

16. Tomato 189

17. Zucchini 176

18. Yellow Squash 150

CHAPTER 5

HYDRATION

Staying hydrated can be a tricky subject when it comes to losing weight for a tournament. There are two common methods of measurement regarding weight loss. One method is body fat weight loss where you create a caloric deficit through diet and daily exercise. The second method that many people confuse with true weight loss is water weight loss through sweat or water weight loss from doing the latest low carbohydrate diet. A wrestler will lose fat weight at an accelerated pace by going through the daily high intensity interval training workouts from their practice. However, there is also the very deceiving water weight loss through sweat from each workout.

A typical day for me in a college wrestling room would be a water weight loss of 4-6 pounds. The combination of intense wrestling workouts in a warm workout room made losing water weight very easy. It is almost guaranteed after 4-6 weeks of rigorous daily weight room workouts, track workouts, and live wrestling caused a significant decrease in body fat weight. For nine years, while coaching at the high school level, I would measure the average body fat loss after an eight-week training program. The average body fat lost was seven pounds after two months of the wrestling season, which included five practices each week and three tournaments each month.

Before every high school season, each wrestler needs to determine the optimum weight class that they will compete in by the winter recess. There will always be a few athletes in the middle of two weight classes. An example would be someone weighing 111 who can bump up to 114 or drop to 108. This is where proper hydration is super important for making the appropriate weight class.

Hydration is key to athletic performance. Studies have shown that exercise performance is impaired when an individual is dehydrated by as little as 2% of body weight. Losses in excess of 5% of body weight can decrease the capacity for work by about 30%. Early signs of dehydration are dry mouth, increased thirst, and dark yellow urine. Bottom line, if you are thirsty you have waited too long to replenish your liquids. You are already dehydrated.

A wrestler who cuts back on complex carbohydrates and water 2-4 days before weigh-ins will feel burnt out physically and mentally. This type of grind-it-out mentality related to the weekly weight cut is one of the main causes for the high turnover rate in high school wrestling.

Many clinical studies have been carried out to explore the effects of dehydration on exercise performance. At 2% water loss or more the following impacts have been observed:

- Dehydration can reduce exercise performance.

- Dehydration can reduce the time to exhaustion.
- Dehydration increases the perception of exercise difficulty.
- Dehydration can reduce mental performance. Therefore alertness, concentration, visual motor skills and decision-making are affected.
- Dehydration and sodium loss can lead to muscle cramps.
- Dehydration is a risk factor for heat exhaustion and heat stroke, both serious conditions.

A good habit to start in the beginning of the season is to routinely check your weight before practice and after practice. Always weigh-in wearing compression shorts or a singlet, which usually weighs (0.4), to get accurate measurement on the digital scale. A daily log of your pre- and post-practice weigh-in is a good indicator of how much water weight is lost in an average practice.

It is also important to be well hydrated prior to practice or competition. This is nearly as important as maintaining that hydration during exercise. To ensure proper pre-exercise hydration, the athlete should consume approximately 500 to 600 ml (17 to 20 fl oz) of water or sports drink 2 to 3 hours before exercise. By hydrating several hours prior to the exercise, there is sufficient time for urine output to return to normal before starting your next workout.

Keep yourself well hydrated.

Water is your body's principal chemical component and makes up about 60 percent of your body weight. Every system in your body depends on water. For example, water flushes toxins out of vital organs, carries nutrients to your cells, and provides a moist environment for ear, nose and throat tissues.

There are many factors affected by water intake: your health, activity, and living environment. When you are dehydrated, your body stores more water for survival, not less. This is where a lot of wrestlers who start cutting out the water in the middle their training cycle get it wrong. This will negatively impact their energy output and performance during practice.

Remember to drink at least nine glasses of water per day. When you get dehydrated, you actually store more water, making the weight cut tougher during the day. Avoid early dehydration in your training cycle, avoid caffeine drinks, and make it a habit to stay hydrated for peak performance.

Hydration Tips:

Drink fluids throughout the day before you exercise. Follow this daily formula.

- Drink 8 ounces of water when you wake up after you weigh-in.
- Drink 8-16 ounces of water or cran-water during brunch or recess period.
- Drink 8-16 ounces of water during lunch or 2 hours before practice.
- 15 minutes before you begin practice, drink between 8-16 ounces of water.
- During your workout, drink another 4 ounces every 15-20 minutes.
- After practice weigh-in drink 8 ounces.
- Before dinner drink 8 ounces of water.

These are the only liquids consumed during the weight cut process. Eliminate all sugary drinks like soda, juice, energy drinks, etc.

Why Cranberry Water?

Adding cranberry water to your daily hydration program can help give you a mild detoxification for your body. Use 100% unsweetened organic cranberry juice. Do not confuse this with the 100% cranberry juice mix variety that can be combined with apple, grape, or other corn syrup ingredients. Blend 2 ounces of 100% unsweetened cranberry juice with 14 ounces of filtered water. Drink 16 ounces of cranberry water daily going into your weigh-in.

A cranberry water blend supports liver function. The organic acids act as digestive enzymes, which help the body remove small fatty deposits from the lymphatic system of the body. Cranberry water also helps flush toxins from foods that are high in sodium, sugar, and fat that causes excess water retention. Finally cranberry water strengthens the immune system, which can be a valuable asset during the flu and cold winter wrestling season.

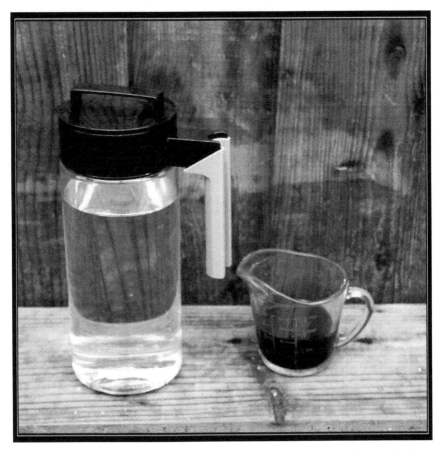

Mix 80% water with 20% pure unsweetened cranberry juice.

Energy Drinks

In 2006, there were more than 30% of adolescents reported using energy drinks. Energy drinks have become a $3.5 billion dollar industry. I don't recommend that athletes rely on energy drinks during their weight cut process because of the excess caffeine that are in the energy drinks. Here are some reasons how caffeine can negatively affect your sports performance:

- The FDA recommends a limit of 65 grams of caffeine per 12 fluid ounces.
- The Cooper Clinic recommends that adults consume less than 200 mg of caffeine a day.
- Energy drinks are not just your usual caffeine and sugar combinations. There are other stimulants added that you should be aware of that can give your teen serious side effects.
- Caffeine acts as a mild diuretic and can lead to dehydration.
- Caffeine causes slight rise in your blood insulin level.
- Recognize the ingredients in energy drinks listed below. They are unregulated and contain harmful additives that intensify the effects of caffeine.
  - Guarana and kola nuts are additional source of caffeine.
  - Bitter orange and citrus aurantium contain synephrine.
  - Ma Huang is a plant source for ephedra.

- o Geranium is a source of methylhexaneamine, which is banned by the NCAA.

- The marketing of these beverages targets young athletes and promises high-energy boost and enhanced focus. Be aware of labels that say, "Pre-game sports drink."
- Read the labels. Example: An energy drink contains 50 mg caffeine per serving. However, you should note that that is only 2 fluid ounces per serving and the drink contains 8.4 ounces. This drink really has over 200 mg of caffeine in a can.
- Wrestling pushes your anaerobic threshold. Relying on high caffeinated energy drinks as a Pre-game sports drink can lead to dehydration and symptoms that can impair performance. Caffeinated beverages can lead to nausea, agitation, and palpitations.

Energy Drinks and Caffeine Content

Product	Size of Drink	Caffeine
Starbucks Brewed Coffee	8 oz	180 mg
Full Throttle	16 oz	144 mg
NOS	16 oz	260 mg
Rock Star	16 oz	160 mg
Red Bull	8.3 oz	80 mg
5 Hour Energy	2 oz	200 mg
Coke	12 oz	51 mg
Diet Coke	12 oz	45 mg
Monster	16 oz	140 mg

CHAPTER 6

KEEPING IT GREEN

A colorful plate full of green leafy vegetables can be a rare sight for many young athletes and weekend warriors. Your weight cut diet should be a combination of fruits, vegetables, beans, healthy whole grains, fish, and lean protein. The emphasis of this "clean" eating plan is to eat healthy, fiber rich, unprocessed foods with a high ORAC value. Keeping it "green and clean" also means hydrating properly with filtered water, drinking cranberry water daily and incorporating green juice or green smoothies. Your body will thank you for eating this way! You will feel the difference in your strength and energy levels!

FIBER

Fiber is found in fruits, whole grains, and beans. The recommended daily amount of fiber for men is 30 grams and 25 grams for women. Teen fiber guidelines are the same as adults. You will have great energy for practice and feel full throughout your day with a fiber rich diet!

There are many other benefits in the fiber-eating plan besides making you feel full and regulating digestion. Fiber is an incredible nutrient that lowers cholesterol, protects your heart health, and aids in weight management. High fiber food can sometimes cause cramps and frequent bathroom breaks during exercise. Make sure you slowly integrate fiber into your diet.

Check out the list of legumes and vegetables below that will provide you with 5-10 grams of fiber per item. This list will help you understand the serving size in order to get 5-10 grams of fiber in each meal. You can meet your daily needs from 3 cups of vegetables, 2 cups of fruit, whole grain or double fiber bread, cereal, and side dishes like quinoa. Always strive to get your fiber requirements for the day.

true walking weight. By following our method, you can focus on practicing hard, burning off unwanted fat, and cutting weight in a safe manner.

In the next chapter we will discuss the old methods often associated with cutting weight. My goal is to change the old mentality and offer a safe alternative to cutting weight for sports. Weight divisions will always challenge individual choices and make you evaluate where you can have the most success. You will learn healthy habits that will help you achieve your weight loss and athletic goals. I encourage parents and relatives of young athletes to join the cutting weight 101 movement and get their weight down to a healthy body fat percentage as well.

<u>Legumes & Vegetables</u> (10 grams in each)

1. 1/2 cup mixed beans or 2 cups soybeans
2. 1 cup split peas or lentils
3. 2 cups of broccoli
4. 3 cups steamed vegetables
5. 1 medium artichokes or 1 cup of peas
6. 1 cup black beans or lima beans
- The darker the color of the vegetable the higher the fiber content. Spinach-7 grams of fiber for 1 cup.

<u>Fruits</u>

1. Raspberries (1 cup) = 8 grams of fiber
2. Pear with skin = 5.5 grams of fiber
3. Apple with skin = 4.4 grams of fiber
4. Guava = (1 cup) 9 grams of fiber
5. Prunes = (½ cup dried) 6.2 grams of fiber
6. Blackberries = (1 cup) 7.6 grams of fiber

Whole Grains

1. Yellow Box Barilla Spaghetti = (1 cup) 6.3 grams of fiber
2. Oatmeal = (1 cup) 4 grams of fiber
3. Brown Rice = (1 cup) 3.5 grams of fiber
4. Organic Quinoa = (1 cup) 12 grams of fiber
5. Whole wheat bread = (1 slice) 3-5 grams of fiber
6. Whole wheat spaghetti = (1 cup) 6-8 grams of fiber

GOING GREEN

One of easiest ways of getting the best nutrients during the week of a weight cut is drinking cold pressed green juices or blended green smoothies. The green drink route is an essential part of the plan. Greens help improve electrolyte function. Electrolytes are minerals like sodium, calcium, potassium, and magnesium that give the body energy, and therefore help sport performance.

Cold pressed green juices are becoming more readily available in stores like Trader Joe's, Whole Foods, and Fresh and Easy. If you prefer to make your own green smoothie, prepping with your blender is simple. Try these green smoothie recipes.

1. **Green Smoothie #1:** 1 cup of organic spinach, ½ avocado, 1 cup organic 100% carrot juice, and juice of ½ a lemon. Blend in your blender for 1 minute. Add ¼ cup water if it is too thick for your liking.

2. **Green Smoothie #2:** 1 cup of organic kale with center vein removed, 1 cup organic 100% carrot juice, ½ cup of frozen organic berries, and juice of ½ a lemon.

3. **Green Smoothie #3:** 1 cup of organic greens mix (arugula, spinach, kale, etc), 1 cup of water, 1 green organic apple, ½ lemon, and 1 inch slice of ginger.

4. **Green Smoothie #4:** 1 cup of organic almond milk, ½ avocado, 1-cup organic spinach, and ½ cup of frozen strawberries.

5. **Green Smoothie #5:** Kale power smoothie at your local juice shop.

6. **Green Juice #6:** Trader Joe's or Whole Foods Cold Pressed Green Juice.

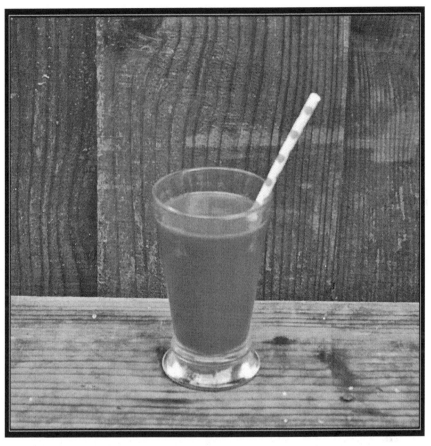

Hydrate with cold pressed green juice daily. Only 100 calories.

Super foods

Feed your cells with premium fuel! Studies have shown that eating super foods with a high ORAC value have great antioxidant benefits. (See Chapter 4 for a super food list with high ORAC value.) They also have the capacity to improve sports performance, reduce muscle damage after exercise, and delay fatigue by neutralizing free radicals!

Super foods contain extremely high-levels of powerful antioxidants. Examples of super foods are goji berries and acai berries, which contain up to 65 times the level of better-known antioxidants like blueberries, blackberries, raspberries, and cranberries. The more antioxidants there are in your diet, the better chance you have of fighting off viruses like the cold and flu and helping your body to fight free radicals. Free radicals damage cells and are produced from intense workouts.

Antioxidant-rich super foods protect cells from damage and repair them to their original, healthy state. Use these super foods in your green smoothies if possible!

Keeping it green 1-2 weeks before your first weigh-in will fill your cells with proper nutrition and antioxidants. This is critical in post-workout recovery, too. Make sure your grocery cart is filled with items from the super foods list for you to use in your smoothies and salads. You will have better muscular endurance and a quicker recovery time when eating prunes, acai berries, blueberries, blackberries, kale, and spinach. Incorporate these healthy snacks during your training cycle.

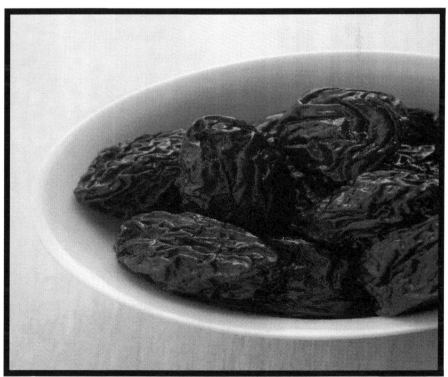

Prunes take time to digest. Try this high fiber snack early in the day.

CHAPTER 7

LOSE FIVE IN FIVE

Now that you know about the benefits of eating clean and green, it's time to give you a plan to follow. There are hundreds of recipes and methods to help you eat healthy and lose weight. This is a simple game plan that will get you down to your fighting weight. Follow my game plan and watch your weight drop. Please do yourself a favor and stay away from eating out and especially fast food while cutting weight. Sound easy? Every champion knows that discipline is the key to any successful endeavor. Follow the game plan and stay focused on creating daily healthy eating habits. You will notice increased energy in practice, tournaments, and peak performance for the post season!

The Game Plan:

1. **MEAL PLAN:** Begin a five-day meal plan the week prior to your Saturday 6am weigh in. (See the sample meal plan later in this chapter.)

2. **HYDRATION: It is very important to stay hydrated throughout the weight cutting process.** A common mistake many athletes make is that they dehydrate their body and lose vital electrolytes, which has a direct effect on energy levels. Do not make this mistake!! Drink at least 64 oz. of filtered water and 16 oz. of cran-water (see chapter 5) each day. Prepare 5 (16 oz. bottles) of cran-water on Monday. Put them in your refrigerator so they are ready to go for the week.

3. **GREEN DRINK:** Make sure you drink at least one green smoothie or cold pressed green juice each day (see chapter 6). The enzymes are very important for your cells and energy. If you can't make your own green smoothie, you can look for cold pressed green juice in your grocery store.

Don't confuse this with the other 100% juice smoothies. Go to Trader Joe's, Whole Foods, or Fresh and Easy to find the cold pressed green juices. Drink your way to an easy and safe weigh-in!

4. **FOOD JOURNAL:** Make sure you journal your food and fluid intake each day (see Chapter 8).

5. **WORKOUT:** Work out every day leading up to weigh-ins. Your average workout time should be 2 hours, burning between 600-1000 calories. Wrestling is a high calorie workout, and this is a typical calorie burn for an average wrestling practice. For non-wrestlers following this plan, it is similar to an hour of cross-fit training followed by a 60 minute Boot camp/High Intensity Interval Training (HIIT)/spin class.

6. **MORNING WEIGHT CHECK:** Check your weight on your home scale first thing each morning to determine your true weight. Don't forget to bring your home scale to practice and compare the difference between the two scales.

To keep everything simple, follow the six steps that I just mapped out, and your weight cut will be very systematic. I have coached many athletes through this process, and my plan really works when done properly.

Next, I will go into detail with two five-day meal plans. First is a real world case study that will show you that you can feel great going into weigh-ins by staying disciplined with your diet, hydration, and workouts. This case study shows some "cheating" junk food early in the training cycle, and hydration was maintained throughout the diet.

Real World Case Study

Case Study: Cutting Weight 101

Starting Weight: 110 lbs. on Sunday morning.
Goal: Need to cut 6 lbs. by Friday afternoon 5pm. Make weight at 104 .lbs by Friday. 5PM weigh-ins.

- Practice in shorts/singlet and t-shirt.
- Thursday, run in sweats to get a good sweat before drilling.
- Maintain water intake early in the week.

Sunday

Morning weight: 110 lbs.

Breakfast: Shake (180 calories/18 grams protein : 1 cup almond milk, 1 scoop raw protein, 1/2 banana)

Brunch: Cliff bar, ½ cup raisins, and cran-water

Lunch: Thanksgiving leftovers: Mac and Cheese

Dinner: Cheeseburger and sweet potato fries

Monday

Morning weight: 109 lbs.

Breakfast: 1 cup Rice Chex and 1/2 cup almond milk

Brunch: Greek yogurt tube

Lunch: 16 oz. cran-water, PBJ sandwich on high fiber bread, 2 tangerines, red grapes.

Dinner: 1 cup gluten-free pasta and 4 turkey meatballs

Tuesday

Morning weight: 108 lbs.

Breakfast: 1 cup grape nuts cereal, sprinkle of brown sugar, 1/2 cup almond milk

Brunch: 16 oz cran-water and 1/4 cup trail mix

Lunch: PB and jelly, ½ cup blueberries, 12 oz. water

Dinner: Rotisserie chicken breast and kale salad

Wednesday

Morning weight: 108 lbs.

Breakfast: 1 cup grape nuts cereal, sprinkle of sugar, 1/2 cup almond milk

Brunch: 16 oz cran-water, apple

Lunch: PB and jelly sandwich, 12 oz. water, sandwich baggie of grapes and ½ cup blueberries

Dinner: corn-on-the-cob, 4 scrambled eggs, 2 tbs. salsa

Thursday

Morning weight: 107.6 lbs.

Breakfast: Shake (180 calories/18 grams protein : 1 cup almond milk, 1 scoop raw protein, 1/2 banana)

Brunch: apple

Lunch: PB sandwich, 16oz. water, 2 tangerines

Workout: 90 min practice. Start w/ 25 min jog in sweats.

Dinner: 16 oz cold pressed green juice (100 calories)

Extra Cardio-workout: 25 min easy on elliptical trainer + 1 mile run

Friday

Morning weight: 104.2 lbs.

Breakfast: 16 oz cold pressed green juice (100 calories)

Brunch: Orange

Lunch: Skip: workout (run 1 mile and drill for 25 minutes).

Drive 2 hours to tournament: Chew gum

Weigh-in: 5PM.

Weight at weigh-ins: 103.6 lbs

After weigh-ins: Hydrate 12 oz. water. Followed by 16oz coconut water for electrolytes.

Dinner: Pasta feed, bread and 16 oz. water.

Saturday: Tournament day

Breakfast: Cold pressed green juice, bagel with peanut butter, banana. Drink 12 oz. of water after each match.

Snacks: Apple, 2 bananas

Lunch: PBJ sandwich

Results: Placed second in national tournament with lots of energy = Peak Performance. Never felt tired or fatigue during the day.

Ideal Five-Day Meal Plan

The ideal meal plan shows a nice balance of high fiber, nutrient dense food, and super food kale smoothies and green juice. This plan will give you high energy the entire week and also emphasizes staying hydrated throughout your training cycle.

Scenario: Joe Bye weighs 157 lbs. He needs to make 152 lbs. for Saturday morning 6AM weigh-in.

<u>Monday</u>

- **Morning Weigh-in:** 157 lbs.
- **Breakfast:** Protein smoothie. 1 cup unsweetened almond milk. 1 banana. 1 scoop raw protein powder. ½ cup of ice. Blend protein smoothie.
- **Lunch:** 1 tablespoon of organic peanut butter. 1 tsp. of organic jelly. 2 slices of double fiber bread. Small baggie of grapes. 1 bottle of Cran-Water. 1 apple.
- **Afternoon or after school snack:** Green Shake #1 (see chapter 6)
- **After Practice Weigh-in:** 155 lbs. (-2 pounds)

- **Dinner/Post Practice:** 6 oz skinned chicken breast. 1-cup brown rice. 1.5 cups of veggies. Broccoli Salad. 2 tbsp. of vinaigrette dressing. 1 cup of hot lemon water.

Tuesday

- **Morning Weigh-in:** 156 lbs.
- **Breakfast:** Scrambled eggs (1 whole, 3 whites). 2 slices whole-wheat toast. 16 oz of water.
- **Lunch:** 1 pear, Turkey sandwich lettuce/tomato, and 1 bottle cran-water.
- **Afternoon or after school snack:** 1 cold pressed Green Juice.
- **After Practice Weigh-in:** 154 lbs. (-2 pounds)
- **Dinner/Post Practice:** Chicken caesar salad. 1 cup of tomato soup. 16 oz. water.

Wednesday

- **Morning Weigh-in:** 155 lbs.
- **Breakfast:** Green Juice.
- **Snack:** 1 apple. 16 oz water.
- **Lunch:** 1 cup blackberries, 1 cup low fat cottage cheese, 1 tbsp almonds.

- **Afternoon or After-school snack:** Zone Perfect bar. 16 oz. water.
- **After Practice Weigh-in:** 153 lbs. (-2 pounds)
- **Dinner/Post Practice:** Vegetable Lasagna. Serving size similar to two hockey pucks.

Thursday

- **Morning Weigh-in:** 154 lbs.
- **Breakfast:** 2-3 hard-boiled eggs.
- **Snack:** Apple and 1 bottle cran-water.
- **Lunch:** 4.5 oz water packed tuna salad, 1 whole-wheat pita pocket.
- **Afternoon or after school:** Cold pressed green juice.
- **After Practice Weigh-in:** Log your weight. 152.4 lbs.
- **Dinner/Post Practice:** 4 oz. baked salmon and 1 cup roasted vegetables.

Friday

- **Morning Weigh-in:** 153 lbs. (By Friday morning, you should be 1-2 pounds away from your weight goal.)
- **Breakfast:** 8 oz. water. Green smoothie.
- **Brunch 10:30am:** 8 oz water.
- **Lunch:** 300-calorie salad and 16 oz. water.
- **Afternoon:** 1 cran-water.
- **After Practice Weigh-in:** 150.8 lbs.
- **Dinner/Post Practice:** Green smoothie.

Friday Night: The Night Before Weigh-ins

The night before a morning weigh-ins is the most important night of the weight cut process. This is where I have seen many wrestlers not make weight and lose an opportunity to compete. Depending upon how much you have to lose on Friday night, I have three different strategies to make weight by Saturday morning.

Know your weight. Make sure you know the difference between your home scale and the calibrated team scale. There is usually a +/- 1-2 pound difference.

You will fall in these three categories. Know your category and stay on track with your Friday night plan.

1. **Lucky category:** You are under 2-4 pounds after practice. You can have salad for dinner instead of green juice.

2. **Cutting it close category:** You are one pound or half a pound under. Play it smart when you are this close to making weight. Stay disciplined and avoid any temptations that will put on quick water weight.

3. **Oh-oh category:** You are 1-3 pounds over your weight class after practice. Rest for 1-3 hours and you will need to go do another cardio workout session that night. It is best to avoid high impact runs/sprints/plyometrics, so you don't burn your legs out for the tournament the next day. Get your sweat started and keep it going strong on an exercise bike, rowing machine, or elliptical trainer.

Whatever category you are in, go to sleep early! Find a good distraction, rest up, and visualize your performance. When you wake up on Saturday morning, check your weight right away. You should be half a pound under your competition weight class. Be aware of the variance between your home scale and the certified tournament scale. Always play it safe and don't eat and drink until after 6am weigh-ins. You can chew gum or have a breath mint to distract you before weigh-ins.

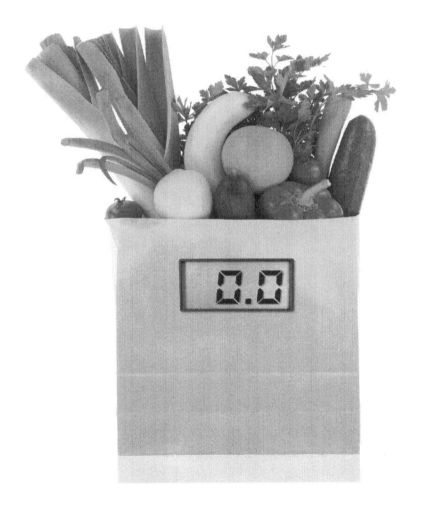

CHAPTER 8

Champion's Journal Goals

Starting a food journal and tracking your calorie intake is a prerequisite for a safe and effective weight loss. Food journals or calorie tracking apps with your smartphone will help with accountability, awareness, and weight loss. Weight loss researchers revealed that tracking your calories coming in can double the amount of weight loss. Consistent daily tracking can be simple and requires no fancy equipment. Just use a pen and paper or a calorie counting app from iTunes or Android platforms and you are on your way to losing fat the right way.

Always carry a notebook. And I mean always. The short-term memory only retains information for three minutes; unless it is committed to paper you can lose an idea for ever.
– Will Self

The most important rule in food journaling is consistent daily calorie intake tracking. You have to write down everything you eat and drink. If you are dedicated toward a healthy weight cut, you will need to write down everything good and bad that you put in your body. Being 100% honest when you input meals in your food journal is a requirement of this program. If you download a calorie-tracking app, the program will identify your daily caloric intake in order to reach your weight loss goal. If you don't want to use an app, you can track the your food and drink calories in a notebook.

Food journaling can be eye-opening and revealing. Your daily eating and drinking habits - the good, the bad, and the ugly - are exposed. When I look at the food journals of my wrestlers and weight loss clients, I can usually see the common habits of not eating enough for breakfast, not drinking enough water, snacking on chips, soda, or juice boxes during lunch, and eating large portion meals for dinner followed by high sugar dessert.

As a wrestler, you work hard in practice and burn hundreds of calories every day. Remember to write down how much you have eaten and the times of the day that you are eating your meals. It is very important to monitor your daily eating habits and make the appropriate changes to help attain peak performance. Small steps in change can lead to more success in making long term changes. After a week of journaling, nutritional habits are exposed. Adding healthy choices will be easier to include in your daily diet.

In order for journaling to be successful in weight loss, the person tracking calories needs to be held accountable by a coach or a parent. In most cases parents establish the eating habits, and having one of your parents take part in the weight loss challenge can be very helpful. It does not help a teenage athlete if their parents bring home fast food or offer to eat out the day before weigh-ins. Your coach should also check your journal a few times a week. Knowing that a coach will look at your food journal will keep you accountable and keep you from grabbing another piece of pizza or drinking another can of soda.

If you plan to get help from both your coach and your parents, it is important for your coach and parents to be on the same page. Open communication between coaches and parents is crucial to successful weight loss. If a wrestler's mom is not in favor of her son going to a lower weight class, then that wrestler should probably bump up a weight class and not worry about losing weight.

When I talk about going down a weight class or cutting weight, I am referring to a 3-5 pound drop from a person that is in the athlete or fitness range of body fat percentage. The fitness range for men is 14-17% and women 21-24%. A successful weight-cutting program includes food journaling and proper hydration. Food journaling breed's discipline and a disciplined wrestler will become a successful student athlete!

Here is a case study of a typical food journal from one of my high school wrestlers:

Date: 1/4/2013.

Day: Monday.

Next Weigh-in: Wednesday Night League Dual Meet.

Breakfast: Nothing

Brunch: Peanut Butter Crackers, Cheese Puffs, and Chocolate Milk.

Lunch: Pizza, Fries, and Soda.

Dinner: Big Cheeseburger, 6 piece nuggets, 16 oz Diet Coke. Dessert: Ice cream bar.

As you can see, he is clearly missing a few healthy choices and the recommended amount of fruits and vegetables in his diet. He can easily add healthy options during breakfast, lunch, and after practice to get the proper fuel for his body. He should stock up on food from the super food orac value list, drink 8-10 glasses of water everyday, and stay committed to his food journal every day of the week. It takes 5 minutes of daily meal planning to make healthy additions to one's diet. An athlete who is 100% committed will get the most desired results.

At the end of this chapter, you will find a few sample journal entries that will give you good ideas for your weight cutting journey. Follow the Weight Cut 101 Journal. Complete the checklist of items to streamline a successful and healthy weight cut. Make sure you journal your morning weight, your daily meals, and your daily goals. Don't forget to drink cran-water and plenty of water daily. The benefits of keeping a weight cut journal will not only help you make weight, it also reinforces discipline and documents important action steps. The Cutting Weight 101 Journal records progress, causes the individual to become intentional and makes their goal appear closer and attainable.

It's difficult staying committed to food journaling every day. Seeing inspirational quotes for daily motivation helps keep the action steps in motion toward a championship lifestyle. Next, you will see samples of the cutting weight 101 lifestyle. Staying hydrated is the common theme in each journal. Make journaling your daily habit!

Sample Cutting Weight 101 Journal
Date: 11/17/14

Journal Items	Notes/Times
Morning Weigh-in	137.8 Pounds (5:40AM)
Breakfast	Scrambled Eggs, 1 slice double fiber bread, 1 Pear (6:50am)
Green Drink	Kale cold pressed juice. 1 bottle (10:30am brunch)
Lunch	4.5 oz chicken breast sandwich on 2 pieces of whole wheat bread. Apple
8 oz. Cran-Water	Noon
Cardio-Weights	Run: 2.5 mile warm-up run/practice 3:30PM
16 oz. Glasses of Water	**1 breakfast, 1 green, 1 cran-water, 8 oz practice, 8 oz after practice**
Skills Drilled/Reps	45 double legs, 45 snaps and go behind, 18 mins live matches.
Post Practice Weight	136.2 pounds
Dinner	5.5oz baked Halibut, 2.5 cups veggies, 1 cup whole wheat pasta
8 oz. Cran- Water	1PM
Daily Goal	Work on snap-post-go's during live. Study for upcoming math test, 11/20.
Monthly Goal	Certify 132 before Thanksgiving. Win Iron Man Tournament
Post Season Goal	Win League, Sections, State, Be an All American/National Champion

Sample Cutting Weight 101 Journal

Date: <u>11/18/14</u>

Journal Items	Notes
Morning Weigh-in	136.4
Breakfast	Fiber One Cereal with Almond milk
Green Drink	Brunch: Kale green cold pressed juice
Lunch	Classic Greek Salad and 4 oz. Chicken Breast.
8 oz. Cran-Water	Drink 8 oz. lunch.
Cardio-Weights	6AM Lift & 3 mile run
16 oz. Glasses of Water	**1 breakfast, 1 green, 1 cran-water, 8 oz practice, 16 oz after practice**
Skills Drilled/Reps	Front Headlock offense, leg riding/defense, 50 Drive Doubles
Post Practice Weight	134.8
Dinner	Lemon Salmon with Lima Beans
8 oz. Cran- Water	Before practice 3:00
Daily Goal	Study for Math Test. Drill in solid stance. Work on shot counters.
Monthly Goal	Certify at 132 pounds. Win Iron Man. Win First Scrimmage.
Post Season Goal	Win Section, State, Be an All American, National Champion

Sample Cutting Weight 101 Journal

Date: 11/19/14

Journal Items	Notes
Morning Weigh-in	135
Breakfast	Raw Protein shake with ½ Banana
Green Drink	Brunch: Kale green cold pressed juice
Lunch	Turkey Sandwich on high fiber bread
8 oz. Cran-Water	Drink 8 oz. lunch.
Cardio-Weights	6AM Lift & 4 (4X40 sprints)
16 oz. Glasses of Water	**1 breakfast, 1 green, 1 cran-water, 8 oz practice, 16 oz after practice**
Skills Drilled/Reps	Front Headlock Defense, Wrist ride/defense, 50 Swing Singles, 3 finishes
Post Practice Weight	134
Dinner	6 oz chicken breast, Quinoa/Veggies
8 oz. Cran- Water	Before practice 3:00
Daily Goal	Do well Math Test, Work on stance and motion the entire practice.
Monthly Goal	Certify at 132 pounds. Win Iron Man. Win First Scrimmage.
Post Season Goal	Win Section, State, Be an All American. National Champion

Sample Cutting Weight 101 Journal

Date: <u>11/20/14</u>

Journal Items	Notes
Morning Weigh-in	134
Breakfast	Fiber One Cereal with Almond milk
Green Drink	Brunch: Kale green cold pressed juice
Lunch	Lemony Kale Salad and 4 oz. Chicken Breast.
8 oz. Cran-Water	Drink 8 oz. lunch.
Cardio-Weights	6AM Drill & 4 mile run
16 oz. Glasses of Water	**1 breakfast, 1 green, 1 cran-water, 8 oz practice, 16 oz after practice**
Skills Drilled/Reps	Front ¼ , leg riding/Turk, 50 Doubles and 50 short sit outs/hip heist
Post Practice Weight	133
Dinner	4 oz lean ground turkey/Pasta/Veggies
8 oz. Cran- Water	Before practice 3:00
Daily Goal	Study Chemistry Test, Drill in Hi-C and finish for 10 minutes after practice.
Monthly Goal	Certify at 132 pounds. Win Iron Man. Win First Scrimmage.
Post Season Goal	Win Section, State, Be an All American. National Champion.

Sample Cutting Weight 101 Journal

Date: <u>11/21/14</u>

Journal Items	Notes
Morning Weigh-in	133.8
Breakfast	Fiber One Cereal with Almond milk
Green Drink	Brunch: Kale green cold pressed juice
Lunch	4 oz pork loin, 2 cups broccoli, 1 cup zucchini, ½ bell pepper.
8 oz. Cran-Water	Drink 8 oz. lunch.
Cardio-Weights	6AM Drill & 25 minute circuit training
16 oz. Glasses of Water	**1 breakfast, 1 green, 1 cran-water, 8 oz practice, 16 oz after practice**
Skills Drilled/Reps	Short offense, leg riding/defense, 50 Inside trips, 30 Stand up escapes
Post Practice Weight	131.8
Dinner	5 oz. Chicken Breast/Brown Rice/Veggies
8 oz. Cran- Water	Before practice 3:00
Daily Goal	Do well Chemistry Test. Drill in low singles 15 minutes after practice.
Monthly Goal	Certify at 132 pounds. Win Iron Man. Win First Scrimmage.
Post Season Goal	Win Section, State, Be an All American. National Champion.

Sample Cutting Weight 101 Journal

Date: <u>11/22/14</u>

Journal Items	Notes
Morning Weigh-in	133.2 (Saturday Practice)
Breakfast	Yogurt /Granola/1 cup raspberries
Green Drink	Brunch: Beets cold pressed juice
Lunch	Vegetable Pot Pie, 9 grape tomotoes.
8 oz. Cran-Water	Drink 8 oz. lunch.
Cardio-Weights	9AM Drill & 35 minute circuit training
16 oz. Glasses of Water	**1 breakfast, 1 green, 1 cran-water, 8 oz practice, 8 oz after practice**
Skills Drilled/Reps	Shrugs, Granby rolls/defense, 50 Tilts, 50 Stand up escapes
Post Practice Weight	131.8
Dinner	4 oz. Chicken Kabob/Pita/Hummus/Veggies
8 oz. Cran- Water	After practice 3:00
Daily Goal	Do History Project. Drill extra knee pull singles 15 minutes after practice.
Monthly Goal	Certify at 132 pounds on 11/29 Win Iron Man. Win First Scrimmage.
Post Season Goal	Win Section, State, Be an All American. National Champion 132 pounds!

Sample Cutting Weight 101 Journal

Date: 11/23/14

Journal Items	Notes
Morning Weigh-in	133 (Sunday/Champions Workout)
Breakfast	Steel Cut Oatmeal with Blueberries
Green Drink	Brunch: Kale Smoothie #3
Lunch	Brown rice/Sweet Sour Chicken
8 oz. Cran-Water	Drink 8 oz. lunch.
Cardio-Weights	8AM 3 mile run. 10 Big Momma Hills
16 oz. Glasses of Water	**1 breakfast, 1 green, 1 cran-water, 8 oz practice, 8 oz after practice**
Skills Drilled/Reps	Stance and motion 6-10 minutes. 100 pull-ups, 100 Push ups in 2 minutes
Post Practice Weight	132
Dinner	Grilled Sea Bass/Arugula Leaves
8 oz. Cran- Water	4pm
Daily Goal	Finish History project. Run 6 minute mile. 10 Hill sprints.
Monthly Goal	Certify at 132 pounds on 11/29. Win Iron Man. Win First Scrimmage.
Post Season Goal	Win Section, State, Be an All American. National Champion.

CHAPTER 9

GET THE EDGE

Do you want to get an edge on your competition? Stay disciplined on the factors that you can control. You can control your mental and physical training, diet, rest and recovery. These are all key elements to a long and successful athletic career. Here are ten healthy tips to help you get the edge on your competition!

1. Don't skip meals.

Skipping meals will only play havoc with your blood sugar levels and program your metabolism to store fat. You may also lose muscle tissue and lower your basal metabolic rate. Make sure to eat breakfast, a brunch snack, and a big lunch before practice. Post practice you should have a dinner that is high in protein and vegetables with a small amount of complex carbohydrates. Please stop skipping meals! Many wrestlers are so hungry that by the time dinner rolls around, they eat everything they can get their hands on! This not only prevents weight loss, but also leads to weight gain. Streamline the weight cutting process by eating clean and green with proper nutrient timing, journaling the food you put in your body, and staying hydrated.

2. Nutrient Timing.

Your post-exercise meal has the potential to maximize a quick muscle recovery, and therefore it should be consumed 30-45 minutes after practice. This is called the metabolic window. Post practice meals should be planned as one of the primary meals of the day. Combine a protein source, a carbohydrate source, and some greens. A good example would be a grilled chicken breast, ½ cup whole-wheat pasta, and some roasted veggies. This will boost glycogen synthesis and induce muscle damage repair. Eating in this metabolic window can lead to recovery in 4-10 hours. If you miss the metabolic window and eat longer than 45 minutes after practice, your muscle recovery can be as long as 24-36 hours.

3. Don't consume more than about 600 calories per meal if you are trying to lose weight.

This is the maximum number of calories that most people can metabolize without storing fat. Eat smaller meals and supplement with healthy snacks. Spread out your meals with several snacks to keep you feeling full and strong.

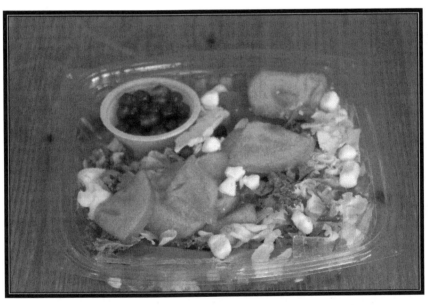

This salad is only 375 calories and very filling.

4. Make sure the fats you consume are healthy.

Healthy fats are an important part of any diet. Fat helps you absorb vitamins and keeps you full. Olive oil is great for salad dressings. I prefer to use avocado and grape seed oil for cooking because they have a higher burning temperature. You don't want your oil to burn when cooking because that can release carcinogens into your food.

When possible, try to get omega-3 fatty acids from foods rather than supplements. Fatty fish is a great way to consume omega-3's. Farm-raised fish of any type may have higher levels of contaminants, so you should choose wild-caught fish when possible. Here are some examples of fatty fish:

- Anchovies
- Bluefish
- Herring
- Salmon
- Sardines
- Sturgeon
- Lake Trout
- Tuna

While foods containing omega-3 fatty acids have health benefits, some -- like oils and nuts -- can be high in calories, so eat them in moderation. I always use the one handful rule. Each handful is about 100-150 calories and one serving (depending on the size of the hand).

5. Read labels to avoid hydrogenated oils.

Many processed foods contain hydrogenated fats and oils. Hydrogenated oils are bad for your health. Avoid foods like crackers, cookies, tortillas and breads when cutting weight. Processed food can be difficult to burn off when they don't provide the proper fuel to meet the high energy demands of aerobic and anaerobic sports. Here are some reasons why processed food can be unhealthy:

1. Processed foods have unhealthy chemical assistance to provide for a long shelf life.
2. Processed foods and sodas are loaded with high sugar and high fructose corn syrup.
3. Junk food and sugar create increased dopamine production in the brain. Food addiction causes over-consumption in low nutrient meals.

6. Avoid saturated fats.

Try to limit your consumption of saturated fats to no more than 10 percent of your fat intake. Calorie counting apps like My Fitness Pal or Lose It can help determine the percentage of saturated fats in your diet. These apps are a great place to food journal while cutting weight. Set yourself up for success by planning ahead and bringing your lunch rather than buying high saturated fat meals from the cafeteria or fast food chains. Brown bag lunches will guarantee better nutrition for your weight cut and will give you more control over unhealthy choices.

7. Use low-fat sources of protein.

Chicken and turkey white meat, fish, low-fat or no-fat cottage cheese, and tofu are excellent sources. Other low fat sources of protein are listed below.

1. Skinless Chicken or Turkey Breast.
2. Flounder, Cod, tuna, and sole.
3. Egg whites.
4. Greek yogurt, cottage cheese, and fat free milk.
5. Beans, peas, and lentils.

8. Sleep is vital.

Sleep is one of the most important ways for the body to recover and regenerate healthy cells. The hormone leptin plays a big role in creating a feeling of satiety. When you don't get enough sleep, your leptin levels drop. You end up feeling tired, hungry, and can crave high-fat and high-calorie foods. Young adults need to develop good sleep habits and getting the recommended 8.5 or 9.25 hours of sleep. Getting enough sleep can help you stay focused and motivated to do well inside and outside the classroom or job. Remember that rest, recovery, and regeneration are just as important as training consistency and intensity.

9. Post-Weigh-In Meal

The post-weigh-in meal can be very large, since most wrestlers have been dieting all week to get their weight down. Many wrestlers plan and dream about their first tasty large meal after weigh-ins. Unfortunately it is very common to see young athletes gulping down sugar-filled energy drinks, and high-fat breakfast food. They tend to stuff themselves with pancakes, bacon and eggs after weigh-ins. The body will fatigue faster during competition because it is working hard to digest the high fat, high sugar influx in the stomach. Many wrestlers have bad first matches because they are dealing with a stomach full of junk food. It's difficult to compete at the top of your game when your body is compromised with bad fuel.

After weigh-ins the body is craving good nutrition that is easy to digest. Remember, you have been eating clean and green for the past two weeks. The last thing you want to do is to put the body into shock with poor fast food choices. Immediately after stepping off the scale, have a green smoothie, water, or an energy drink low in sugar. Your body will thank you for it and your energy during the tournament will be through the roof!

10. Visualize your goals.

A goal is a dream with a deadline. The daily practice of writing down your goals, visual mental rehearsal, and giving yourself a timeline will streamline action steps for achieving your goals. Set aside ten minutes in your day for journaling and practicing deep breathing and imagining how you want your day to progress toward attaining your goals. You will develop daily action steps that will build toward your weekly goals, and ultimately leading to your long-term dream goals. Success is 20% following our cutting weight 101 formula and 80% staying consistent with your daily habits. Everyone will have a different journey in reaching his or her weight loss goals, athletic goals, and life goals. Make your imprint in your journey and don't be afraid to make a commitment to yourself. Follow this cookbook and make weight the correct way. Enjoy the process and embrace the journey of who you become when you reach your ultimate goal.

Sport is quite a simple thing. It is play, and in play, people of all ages find the chance to engage their most profound emotions--love, fear, excitement, disappointment, anger and joy.
- Timothy Shriver, Ph.D.

Made in the USA
Middletown, DE
25 November 2019

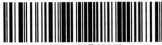

79380588R00068